Skinny Thinking
Chew on This!

Skinny Thoughts and Recipes

For Healthy, Happy Living

Skinny Thinking
Chew on This!

Skinny Thoughts and Recipes

For Healthy, Happy Living

Laura Katleman

Cave of the Heart Publishing

Cave of the Heart Publishing

ISBN:

CONTENTS

Quick, Easy Meals Made with Prepared Sauces   69

Desserts 102

ACKNOWLEGEMENTS

To Gina Lake for your clarity, support, and friendship.

INTRODUCTION

For the past year readers, clients, and workshop participants have been asking me to share some easy to prepare, healthy recipes. I finally sat down with my notebooks and computer files to start writing when a friend called. I told him what I was up to and he suggested interspersing some excepts from the Skinny Thinking book with the recipes—a daily thought on one page and a recipe on the opposite page and voila, the concept for *Chew on This* was born.

My only disclaimer is this: if you are a gourmand for whom the notion of using prepared sauces is tantamount to heresy, this is probably not the cookbook for you. My recipes include prepared sauces whenever possible (from Whole Foods and Trader Joes) for a reason.

It's not just that I'm lazy, though that's part of it. It's not just that I'm trying to save time, though that's part of it. I'm a former food addict who is has ended her love affair with food (although we have remained friends) and as part of the divorce settlement, I consciously chose to lessen my involvement with food. Simply put, I realized that I need to stop living in the kitchen.

If food has been the love of your life, I suggest you consider a similar arrangement. You can still enjoy food and cooking and your kitchen but if you want to heal your misalignment with food, you need to stop spending so much time playing with it in the kitchen.

On the other hand, if you think ovens are metal sweater storage contraptions, saucepans are for bonking unwanted home intruders, and your meals to date have all come in wrappers, let me be the first to introduce you to your kitchen. This is a good starter book for you. If you can read and pour sauce from a jar, you're home free.

Getting Started

Eating healthy and with very little preparation time requires a bit of planning. For example, I always have hard boiled eggs and baked potatoes on hand. With these two ingredients on hand, you have eliminated the most time intensive aspect of making Cobb, chef, and Nicoise salads in one fell swoop! You also have any baked potato meals and your breakfasts-on-the-go virtually done.

And they are so easy to prepare. When you are doing watching television or sorting the laundry just throw 8 baked potatoes in an 350 degree oven and 8 eggs in boiling salted water and set the timer for 15 minutes. When goes it goes off, empty the eggs into the sink and reset the timer for 45 minutes. And viola, there you have the backbone of umpteen healthy meals.

Breakfast

Breakfast on the Go

Organic Instant Oatmeal in a reusable hot cup and a hard boiled egg. I always keep at least a half a dozen hard boiled eggs in my refrigerator in case I need to eat on the run.

Preparation time:
2 minutes if you boil the egg ahead of time.

Nutritional Info:
Servings Per Recipe: 1
Amount Per Serving
Calories: 277.5
Total Fat: 9.3 g
Cholesterol: 212.0 mg
Sodium: 69.1 mg
Total Carbs: 38.6 g
Dietary Fiber: 6.0 g
Protein: 14.3 g

Ingredients:
Quaker Instant Oatmeal, Organic, Regular, 2 serving
Water, tap, 12 fl oz
Hard Boiled Egg, 1 large
1 t. Cinnamon
.25 t. nutmeg

Directions:
Cover the egg in cold water and bring to a boil. Boil the egg for 15 minutes in salted water. Remove rinse with cool water, peel, and eat. Pour contents of instant oatmeal packet into a hot drink cup, add boiling water, stir, let set for a few moments, drink.

Freedom is your birthright!

Know that it is possible to be free from your obsession with food and body weight! It is possible to live without worrying about what you will eat next and whether it will make you fat, or if you'll have the willpower to eat in a way that keeps you from busting out of your jeans. It is possible to free yourself from troubles with food that cause a myriad of health problems, including weight gain. It is possible to live without measuring your self-worth by the vicissitudes of the bathroom scale. It is possible to leave this seemingly insurmountable source of suffering behind.

The most important step in your journey is your decision that you don't want to suffer anymore. You have to say "Enough already!" Then you're ready to find a way out.

Healing means wanting freedom more than you want your old habits.

Raisin Sauce

A great, healthy condiment for oatmeal!

Preparation time:
5 minutes, not counting soaking time.

Nutritional Info:
Servings Per Recipe: 8
Amount Per Serving
Calories: 46.4
Total Fat: 0.1 g
Cholesterol: 0.0 mg
Sodium: 2.7 mg
Total Carbs: 12.2 g
Dietary Fiber: 0.6 g
Protein: 0.5 g

Ingredients:
Raisins, 0.75 cup, packed
Water, tap, 1.50 cup (8 fl oz)

Directions:
Soak raisins in water in an airtight refrigerator for two days. Blend mixture until smooth.

Waking Up Out of the Ego's Relationship with Food

When you are aligned with the ego, you may overeat or eat the wrong foods because your uninvestigated thoughts are mediating between food and you. The ego tempts you with a thin sliver of truth, the pleasurable aspect of eating, and filters out everything else. Then, based on this slant, it creates desires and drives that interfere with a simple and natural relationship with food. Those desires and drives impel you to reach for food whether you're hungry or not, and before you know it, the pounds are piling on.

When you're able to drop out of the ego and move into alignment with the Wise Witness, you're able to see a pure, practical way of eating that's based on food's true function.

The Wise Witness's way of relating to food includes the entire picture—"the whole truth about food."

Huevos Con Verdura

Preparation time:
15-20 minutes

Nutritional Info:
Servings Per Recipe: 2
Amount Per Serving
Calories: 228.1
Total Fat: 10.6 g
Cholesterol: 425.0 mg
Sodium: 437.6 mg
Total Carbs: 19.1 g
Dietary Fiber: 4.1 g
Protein: 15.3 g

Ingredients:
Egg, fresh, 4 large
Salsa, 0.50 cup
Red Ripe Tomatoes, 2 plum tomatoes
Onions, raw, 1 cup, chopped
Garlic, 2 cloves
Carrots, raw, .5 cup, chopped
Cooking Spray

Directions:
Heat a nonstick skillet coated with cooking spray over a medium heat. Sauté onions, garlic, and carrots for a few minutes until soft. Add tomatoes eggs and salsa, stirring until most of the liquid is absorbed. Serve.

Stop Listening to Ego-based Thoughts!

You can become free from ego-based distortions and overblown desires by not listening to the thoughts that create them and by seeing them for what they are, conditioning that keeps us imprisoned in egoic consciousness and suffering.

Your suffering over food and weight has brought you to an exciting watershed in your evolution: realizing that your ego has been lying to you for years. Your willingness to see the truth about how the ego has lied to you what food can give you is what makes permanent healing a real possibility and turns a wonderfully hopeful new page in the story of your journey.

Scrambled Eggs with Tempeh, Salsa, and Cheese

Preparation time:
15 minutes

Nutritional Info:
Servings Per Recipe: 2
Amount Per Serving
Calories: 295.7
Total Fat: 14.3 g
Cholesterol: 428.5 mg
Sodium: 978.0 mg
Total Carbs: 15.6 g
Dietary Fiber: 5.0 g
Protein: 25.3 g

Ingredients:
Egg, fresh, 4 large
Cheddar or Colby Cheese, Low Fat, 0.25 cup, diced
Salsa, 0.50 cup
Fakin' Bacon, 6 strips
Cooking Spray

Directions:
Heat a nonstick skillet coated with cooking spray over a medium heat. Brown Fakin bacon on both sides. Remove and cut into one inch strips. Respray pan, add eggs, salsa, cheese and Fakin bacon, stirring constantly until eggs firm up and liquid is absorbed. Serve.

Enough Already!

The most important step in your journey is your decision that you don't want to suffer anymore. You have to say "Enough already!" Then you're ready to find a way out.

Appetizers

World's Best Guacamole & Chips

Or that's what people tell me anyway!

Guacamole

Nutritional Info:
Servings Per Recipe: 4
Amount Per Serving
Calories: 94.1
Total Fat: 8.1 g
Cholesterol: 0.0 mg
Sodium: 180.2 mg
Total Carbs: 6.2 g
Dietary Fiber: 3.9 g
Protein: 1.3 g

Ingredients:
Avocados, 1
Onions, raw, .25 cup, chopped
Red Ripe Tomatoes, .25 cup, chopped or sliced
Salt, .25 tsp
Pepper, black, 1 dash

Baked Blue Corn Tortilla Chips

Ingredients:
Trader Joes Low Fat Baked Blue Corn Tortilla Chips

Nutritional Info:
Servings Per Recipe: 1
Amount Per Serving
Calories: 110.0
Total Fat: 2.0 g
Cholesterol: 0.0 mg
Sodium: 160.0 mg
Total Carbs: 22.0 g
Dietary Fiber: 2.0 g
Protein: 3.0 g

Directions:
Heat the chips in the oven or toaster oven at 275 degrees for 5-7 minutes. Mash avocado, mix in the rest of the ingredients. Season to taste. Serve

Be Kind to Yourself

If you find yourself following a food thought, be gentle with yourself. We're programmed to listen to and believe our thoughts.

Be kind with yourself about having a food issue. Look around you. Most people have challenging relationships with food. In the case of food and weight, our egoic mind pits two stubborn, mutually exclusive desires against each other: the desire to experience taste pleasure from food and the desire look good. No wonder we're in a pickle! On the one hand, our bodies need food to survive and we're programmed to adore food. On the other hand, we're bombarded with media images of young, thin, attractive people and brainwashed into thinking that we should look that way, too.

Never chastise yourself for having a food issue. The good news is that the food and weight issues that have been the bane of your existence are also your custom-designed ticket to freedom.

A Simple Pragmatic Relationship with Food

How do you relate to food? As a lover, a friend, a god, an enemy, a source of nutrition? What is your image of yourself in relationship to food? What are the thoughts and self-images that mediate between you and food? When you remove all of the thoughts and images that mediate between you and food, what's left? Just a simple, pragmatic relationship with food. That is the goal of *Skinny Thinking*: to help you develop a simple, pragmatic relationship with food.

Easy Caprese

This is an impressive looking appetizer that takes about 5-10 minutes to prepare!

Nutritional Info:
Servings Per Recipe: 8
Amount Per Serving
Calories: 151.0
Total Fat: 10.1 g
Cholesterol: 26.3 mg
Sodium: 216.4 mg
Total Carbs: 3.9 g
Dietary Fiber: 0.7 g
Protein: 11.5 g

Ingredients:
Mozzarella Cheese, part skim milk, 16 oz, sliced
Freshly Ground Black Pepper
Basil, 24 leaves, washed
Extra Virgin Olive Oil, 2 T
Red Ripe Tomatoes, 3 large whole (3" dia), sliced
Coarse Sea Salt

Directions:
Place tomato slices on a platter in a circle. Top each tomato slice with a slice of mozzarella and a basil leaf. Drizzle with olive oil and finish with salt and pepper. Serve.

Healing Food Issues

Ultimately, you must begin to let go of deluded, misguided beliefs and your romanticized relationship with food in order to stop suffering and yo-yoing. In my experience, the best tool to achieve this is inquiry. What is your mental relationship with food. What does it mean to you?

A bird needs both of its wings to fly, and healing your food issues requires both of these two components to be complete and lasting—a shift in your diet and a change in your relationship with food.

Salad Nicoise (Vegetarian Option)

Only 15 minutes to prepare if you use a bottled dressing and cook the eggs and bake the potato ahead of time. I like to keep a supply of both in my refrigerator because they enable me to through together a nutritious meal salad in minutes!

Nutritional Info:
Servings Per Recipe: 2
Calories: 244.0
Total Fat: 6.3 g
Cholesterol: 224.8 mg
Sodium: 307.6 mg
Total Carbs: 25.7 g
Dietary Fiber: 5.7 g
Protein: 23.1 g

Nutritional Info:(vegetarian)
Servings Per Recipe: 2
Calories: 294.7
Total Fat: 8.9 g
Cholesterol: 212.0 mg
Sodium: 634.0 mg
Total Carbs: 35.7 g
Dietary Fiber: 9.7 g
Protein: 20.3 g

Ingredients:
Hard Boiled Egg, 2 large
Pepper, black, 1 dash
Green Beans (snap), 1 cup
Baked Potato (baked potatoes), 1 potato (2-1/3" x 4-3/4")
Spinach, fresh, 8 cups
Tuna, Canned in Water, 3 oz (vegetarian option substitute LightLife Fakin' Bacon 6 strips (browned on the stovetop))

Directions:
Chop baked potato, break up tuna (or chop Fakin' Bacon), slice the hard boiled egg. Place spinach on a serving platter and arrange all other ingredients artfully on top. Sprinkle with dressing.

Nicoise Dressing

Nutritional Info:
Servings Per Recipe: 3
Amount Per Serving
Calories: 85.7
Total Fat: 9.0 g
Cholesterol: 0.0 mg
Sodium: 116.2 mg
Total Carbs: 1.1 g
Dietary Fiber: 0.1 g
Protein: 0.1 g

Ingredients:
Pepper, black, 1 dash
Salt, 1 dash
Capers, canned, 0.50 tbsp, drained
Olive Oil, 2 tbsp
Garlic, 1 clove
Grey Poupon Dijon Mustard, 0.50 tsp
Balsamic vinegar, 1 tablespoon
Capers Brine, 1 ounce

Letting Go of the Child's False Story

Listening to and following the dictates of the Child is a habit that has grown stronger through years of repetition and reinforcement. But if you believe that breaking this habit is daunting, just remember—you created it in the first place, so you have the power to uncreate it. Of course, the ego wants you to view the desire to experience the taste pleasure of food as impossible to resist because that keeps you from challenging the ego's authority. But now is the time to let go of this false story that you've created.

Goat Cheese and Chicken Salad with Roasted Pear and Walnuts

This is a really tasty salad! If you like a tablespoon or two of Trader Joe's Champagne Pear Vinaigrette With Gorgonzola. It's only 45 calories for 2 Tablespoons!

Nutritional Info:
Servings Per Recipe: 4
Calories: 323.8
Total Fat: 14.2 g
Cholesterol: 73.4 mg
Sodium: 189.4 mg
Total Carbs: 16.7 g
Dietary Fiber: 4.4 g
Protein: 35.0 g

Nutritional Info:
Servings Per Recipe: 4
Amount Per Serving
Calories: 294.0
Total Fat: 15.8 g
Cholesterol: 5.0 mg
Sodium: 582.7 mg
Total Carbs: 26.7 g
Dietary Fiber: 8.4 g
Protein: 15.8 g

Ingredients:
Chicken Breast, no skin, 2 breast, bone and skin removed or Fakin' Bacon, chopped
Pears, fresh, 2 cup sliced
Spinach, fresh, 8 cups
Black Walnuts, 0.50 cup, chopped
Silver Goat Garlic & Herb Goat Cheese, 2 oz

Directions: Toss all ingredients together.

You Are More Powerful Than Your Conditioning

Realize that you are kingmaker and you have the power to debunk your story and withdraw your misguided projections about food. The power of choice has always rested in you. Dethrone food by changing the way you think about. It's just nice tasting nutrition, not your lover, your friend, your main source of comfort or life's greatest pleasure.

If the Child is tempting you with pleasure food and you're not hungry, ask yourself: "What am I telling myself that's creating the impulse to reach for food? What am I thinking? What am I feeling right now?" Then ask yourself if eating the pleasure food will truly satisfy that impulse. Will it alleviate the feeling? Will it solve the problem that you're ruminating over? Will it rewrite history or alleviate worries about the future? Will it allow you to say the things you wanted to say in that conversation with your coworker or spouse or child? What will two minutes with that particular food give you? Are the negative consequences of shame, blame, self-castigation, lethargy, ill health, and weight gain worth it?

Cobb Salad

Nutritional Info:

Servings Per Recipe: 8
Amount Per Serving
Calories: 321.1
Total Fat: 18.4 g
Cholesterol: 143.2 mg
Sodium: 1,161.4 mg
Total Carbs: 21.3 g
Dietary Fiber: 6.8 g
Protein: 20.9 g

Nutritional Info:
(vegetarian)

Servings Per Recipe: 8
Amount Per Serving
Calories: 351.6
Total Fat: 19.4 g
Cholesterol: 131.0 mg
Sodium: 1,166.2 mg
Total Carbs: 26.9 g
Dietary Fiber: 9.7 g
Protein: 23.6 g

Ingredients:
Avocados, 1 fruit without skin and seeds
Onions, raw, 2 cup, sliced
Vegetables, Mixed Salad Greens, 8 serving(s)
Fakin' Bacon, 4 serving
Sliced Turkey Breast, 8 ounces or Quorn Chikn Tenders,
6 servings
Chickpeas (garbanzo beans), .5 cup
Hard Boiled Egg, 4 large
*gorgonzola cheese, 8 oz
Carrots, raw, 1 cup, grated
Red Ripe Tomatoes, 1 cup cherry tomatoes
Black Olives, 16 jumbo diced

Yogurt Salad Dressing

Nutritional Info:

Servings Per Recipe: 8
Amount Per Serving
Calories: 16.6
Total Fat: 0.0 g
Cholesterol: 0.0 mg
Sodium: 26.4 mg
Total Carbs: 1.4 g
Dietary Fiber: 0.0 g
Protein: 2.6 g

Ingredients:
Lemon Juice, 0.50 fl oz
Fresh Chives, 1 tbsp chopped
Parsley, 1 tbsp
Grey Poupon Dijon Mustard, 1 tsp
Fage Greek Yogurt 0% fat, 8 oz

Low Fat Ranch Dressing

Nutritional Info:
Servings Per Recipe: 16
Amount Per Serving
Calories: 17.9
Total Fat: 0.0 g
Cholesterol: 0.0 mg
Sodium: 30.4 mg
Total Carbs: 1.7 g
Dietary Fiber: 0.0 g
Protein: 2.6 g

Ingredients:
Cider Vinegar, 2 tbsp
Lemon Juice, 1 fl oz
Fresh Chives, 2 tbsp chopped
Garlic, 1 clove (remove)
Shallots, 1.50 tbsp chopped
Grey Poupon Dijon Mustard, 1.50 tsp
Fage Greek Yogurt 0% fat, 16 oz
Worcestershire Sauce, 2 serving

Am I Hungry?

Remember to ask yourself if you are hungry before you eat today. Eating when you're not hungry creates a cycle of suffering: You eat to get happy, feel bad for indulging, and then eat more to escape your emotional discomfort.

Don't feel bad for having body and eating issues. They can actually help us see our way to a happier life once we realize that the way we've been thinking and living doesn't serve us. The stressful issues that dog us year after year are most instrumental in catalyzing our growth. Even though they hurt like heck, they're ultimately our ticket to freedom from suffering.

Suffering moves us to break free from our unconscious patterns and conditioning and instead live from the true self. In this state, we are free to experience the peace and joy available in each moment. This is the battle: resistance versus acceptance; the ego versus the true self; self-delusion versus truth; the ego's small sliver of truth about food and the body versus the whole picture.

Honeydew and Avocado Chicken Salad with Fresh Herb Dressing

Nutritional Info:
Servings Per Recipe: 8
Amount Per Serving
Calories: 324.2
Total Fat: 12.0 g
Cholesterol: 51.3 mg
Sodium: 334.1 mg
Total Carbs: 28.0 g
Dietary Fiber: 6.6 g
Protein: 28.2 g

Nutritional Info:
(vegetarian)
Servings Per Recipe: 8
Amount Per Serving
Calories: 286.8
Total Fat: 12.4 g
Cholesterol: 0.0 mg
Sodium: 569.1 mg
Total Carbs: 34.8 g
Dietary Fiber: 9.6 g
Protein: 15.3 g

Ingredients:
Chicken Breast, no skin, 3 breast, bone and skin removed (remove)
Vegetables, Mixed Salad Greens, 8 serving(s)
Honeydew Melon, 1 melon (6" - 7" dia)
Onions, raw, 2 cup, sliced
Avocados, California (Haas), 2 fruit without skin and seeds (remove)
Fakin' Bacon, 4 serving
*Pine Nuts, .5 cup

Herb Parsley Dressing

Nutritional Info:
Servings Per Recipe: 10
Amount Per Serving
Calories: 100.4
Total Fat: 10.8 g
Cholesterol: 0.0 mg
Sodium: 234.6 mg
Total Carbs: 1.3 g
Dietary Fiber: 0.2 g
Protein: 0.2 g

Ingredients:
Olive Oil, .5 cup
Cider Vinegar, .25 cup
Salt, 1 tsp (remove)
Apple juice, unsweetened, .12 cup
Pepper, black, 1 tsp
dry mustard, 1 serving
Garlic, 2 cloves minced
Fresh Parsley, .5 cup minced
Fresh Basil, 3 tbsp

Dressing Directions:
Blend all ingredients

Salad Directions: Spray a skillet with cooking spray. Brown
the chicken breasts (or chik'n tenders). Place a washed
salad greens on a platter. Thinly slice the chicken.
Artfully place the melon, chicken, honeydew, onion,
avocado, fakin' bacon on the platter in that order. Drizzle
with dressing and top with pine nuts.

Ignoring the Voice of the Child

When it comes to food, the pleasure-seeking Child causes us to gain weight by telling us things like "You've been working so hard, you deserve a slice...or two...or three of cheesecake."; "You should live a little. Give yourself a treat."; "Eating a bit more won't hurt."; "You've had a lousy day, so why not make yourself feel better with a little pleasure food?"; and "Indulge now and worry about tomorrow tomorrow."

The Child creates our eating problem by tempting us to use pleasure food as a treat, cajoling us to eat a few more bites even when our stomachs are bursting. Then, the Critic has the unmitigated gall to shame and castigate us over the weight gain the Child caused!

Chicken Tostada Salad

Nutritional Info:

Servings Per Recipe: 4
Amount Per Serving
Calories: 355.0
Total Fat: 3.8 g
Cholesterol: 71.9 mg
Sodium: 536.4 mg
Total Carbs: 35.1 g
Dietary Fiber: 11.9 g
Protein: 46.2 g

Nutritional Info: (vegetarian)

Servings Per Recipe: 4
Amount Per Serving
Calories: 294.1
Total Fat: 2.3 g
Cholesterol: 3.5 mg
Sodium: 676.4 mg
Total Carbs: 42.0 g
Dietary Fiber: 14.8 g
Protein: 27.8 g

Ingredients:
Cheddar or Colby Cheese, Low Fat, 0.50 cup, diced (remove)
Chili powder, 1 tsp
Pepper, black, 1 dash
Salt, 1 dash
Salsa, 1 cup
Onions, raw, 1 cup, chopped
Red Ripe Tomatoes, 1 cup, chopped or sliced
Beans, black, 2 cups
Fage Greek Yogurt 0% fat, 6 oz
Romaine Lettuce (salad), 8 cup, shredded
Chicken Breast, no skin, 2 breast, bone and skin removed or Lightlife Smart Crumbles (Mexican Style)

You Are the Kingmaker!

But how do you break the habit of turning to food in your time of need or celebration or longing? The answer is: Take another look. Open yourself to a broader perspective and come to see the whole truth about food rather than just hanging on to your habitual, unquestioned assumptions.

In your moment of wanting a pleasure food, nothing seems clearer or more powerful than your desire. In those moments, the Child is powerful; she has your undivided attention and it takes tremendous will to say "Not now, dear, maybe later," just as you might to a child who wants a snack right before dinner.

Listening to and following the dictates of the Child is a habit that has grown stronger through years of repetition and reinforcement. But if you believe that breaking this habit is daunting, just remember—you created it in the first place, so you have the power to uncreate it. Of course, the ego wants you to view the desire to experience the taste pleasure of food as impossible to resist because that keeps you from challenging the ego's authority. But now is the time to let go of this false story that you've created.

Realize that you are kingmaker and you have the power to debunk your story and withdraw your misguided projections about food. The power of choice has always rested in you. Dethrone food by changing the way you think about. It's just nice tasting nutrition, not your lover, your friend, your main source of comfort or life's greatest pleasure.

Chinese Cabbage Salad with Chicken(Tofu)

Nutritional Info:
- Servings Per Recipe: 6
- Amount Per Serving
- Calories: 222.6
- Total Fat: 8.7 g
- Cholesterol: 45.6 mg
- Sodium: 760.6 mg
- Total Carbs: 15.4 g
- Dietary Fiber: 3.8 g
- Protein: 22.5 g

Nutritional Info:(vegetarian)
- Servings Per Recipe: 6
- Amount Per Serving
- Calories: 236.1
- Total Fat: 12.8 g
- Cholesterol: 0.0 mg
- Sodium: 949.5 mg
- Total Carbs: 19.4 g
- Dietary Fiber: 5.8 g
- Protein: 13.3 g

Ingredients:
Cider Vinegar, 4 tbsp
Sesame Oil, 2 tbsp
Chicken Breast, no skin, 2 breast, bone and skin removed or baked teriyaki tofu (White Wave or other brand)
Apple juice, unsweetened, 4 fl oz
Cabbage, red, fresh, 1 head, medium (about 5" diameter)
Sesame Seeds, 4 tbsp
Soy sauce (tamari), 4 tbsp

Directions:
Bake or sauté chicken breasts (with a little water in the pan). Cover to cook through. Shred cabbage and blanch for 15 seconds in hot water. Chop chicken or chop tofu. Blend all ingredients and serve. Refrigerate and serve.

See Food for What it Always Has Been—Not a God—Just Food with a Lowercase "F."

Once you've seen the whole truth about food, you can't believe in it or idolize it in the same way. This inexorably changes you and sets the stage for a new, pragmatic, rational relationship with food.

If you notice an urge to eat something when you're not hungry, you're probably involved in a story—something negative that the mind is telling you about yourself, life, others, or something you're doing. At those moments, you're arguing with reality, resisting the way life is showing up.

The habit of eating pleasure food to change your experience, to escape and entertain yourself rather than nourish your body, is an innocent way of trying to love and soothe yourself when your bored or under stress. There's no reason to make yourself feel bad or wrong about this.

Quinoa Chicken (Tempeh) Salad with Raisins. Walnuts & Kale

Nutritional Info:
Servings Per Recipe: 6
Amount Per Serving
Calories: 312.0
Total Fat: 9.1 g
Cholesterol: 45.6 mg
Sodium: 416.8 mg
Total Carbs: 34.4 g
Dietary Fiber: 5.8 g
Protein: 25.6 g

Nutritional Info: (vegetarian)
Servings Per Recipe: 6
Amount Per Serving
Calories: 325.5
Total Fat: 11.1 g
Cholesterol: 0.0 mg
Sodium: 835.7 mg
Total Carbs: 44.4 g
Dietary Fiber: 9.8 g
Protein: 15.5 g

Ingredients
*Ancient Harvest Traditional Whole Grain Quinoa, 1 serving
=.25 cup dry, 1 cup
Water, tap, 1.75 cup (8 fl oz)
Walnuts, .25 cup, chopped
*Kale, cooked, boiled, drained, with salt, 6 cup, chopped
Cinnamon, ground, 1 tbsp
Salt, 1 dash
Pepper, black, 1 dash
Raisins, .25 cup (not packed)
*Extra Light Olive Oil, 1 tbsp
Chicken Breast, no skin, 2 breast, bone and skin removed or
Fakin' Bacon

Directions:
Bring water to a boil in a sauté pan. Add quinoa. Reduce heat and
cover. Allow to simmer until all liquid is absorbed. Sauté chicken
breasts in a little water. cover to cook through.
Chop and blanch kale. Add a dash of salt and pepper. Add
walnuts, cinnamon, and raisins to cooked quinoa. Shred cooked
chicken breast (brown and chop tempeh). To serve, spread Kale
on a platter top with quinoa. Place chicken on top. Drizzle with
olive oil and a dash of salt and pepper.

Is There Something Off that I Need to Address?

One of the costs of overindulging in pleasure food is that it prevents you from experiencing or inquiring about what you're feeling or believing that caused you to want to eat.

The Child goes after pleasure as a way of coping with what it doesn't like about life. When you automatically indulge and fulfill a desire, you miss out on its real message: There's something that's off here that I need to address, either inside myself, in my life, or with another person. Keep this in mind and notice when the Child starts talking to you. Ask yourself, "Is there something that I'm resisting about life, something that I'm trying to cope with by seeking pleasure? Why do I need pleasure now? What do I really need?"

Skinny Greek Salad

Nutritional Info:
Servings Per Recipe: 2
Amount Per Serving
Calories: 177.7
Total Fat: 7.8 g
Cholesterol: 14.9 mg
Sodium: 695.8 mg
Total Carbs: 16.0 g
Dietary Fiber: 2.8 g
Protein: 12.0 g

Ingredients:
Cottage Cheese, 1% Milkfat, 4 oz
Feta Cheese, 1 oz
Romaine Lettuce (salad), 2 cup, shredded
Onions, raw, 0.50 medium (2-1/2" dia)
Spinach, fresh, 4 cup
Kalamata, Green Olives, pitted, 1 oz
Tomato, grape (3oz = approx. 12 tomatoes), 6 oz

Directions:
Chop or slice the onion thin. Crumble the feta. Chop the olives. Poor some of the water from the jar of olives into the bowl and toss all of the ingredients together.

Bring More Awareness to Your Eating

Slow down and notice what happens during a meal. When you first sit down, assuming you're hungry, the first few bites taste delicious. But as you move toward satiation, the experience changes, the law of diminishing returns sets in, and each successive bite becomes less pleasurable. Once you're satiated, the pleasure drops off even faster, until each additional bite becomes downright unpleasant!

Pureed Lentil, Squash, & Vegetable Soup

Nutritional Info

Servings Per Recipe: 10
Amount Per Serving
Calories: 231.4
Total Fat: 3.5 g
Cholesterol: 5.0 mg
Sodium: 711.7 mg
Total Carbs: 31.7 g
Dietary Fiber: 8.1 g
Protein: 21.2 g

Ingredients:
Butternut Squash, 2 cup, cubes
Newman's Own Vodka Sauce, 1/2 cup, 1.5 cup
Peas, frozen, 2 cup
Split Peas, 1 cup
Lentils, 1 cup
Broccoli, frozen, 1 package (10 oz)
Canned Tomatoes, 1 cup
Garlic powder, 1 tbsp
*Onion powder, 1 tbsp (
Salt, .5 tsp
Pepper, black, .5 tsp
Onions, raw, 1 cup, chopped
Quorn Meatless Balls, 10 serving
Water, tap, 4 cup (8 fl oz)

Can I absolutely know that this is true?

If you uncover a belief or story that causes you to feel bad and overeat, like a good prosecutor, begin to gather evidence to support the veracity of your belief. Is the story you're telling yourself true? If you're going to believe something and let it ruin your mood and run your life, shouldn't it at least be true? As a reasonable, rational person, shouldn't that be your minimum requirement?

When you are tied up in a negative story, ask yourself, "Can I absolutely know that this is true? Can I know that I shouldn't have to do this task? Is it really true that I'm always making a mess of things or that so-and-so is always busting my chops?"

Easy Peasy Split Pea Soup

Nutritional Info:
Servings Per Recipe: 6
Amount Per Serving
Calories: 96.5
Total Fat: 0.3 g
Cholesterol: 0.0 mg
Sodium: 1,564.0 mg
Total Carbs: 17.7 g
Dietary Fiber: 5.5 g
Protein: 5.5 g

Ingredients:
Pepper, black, 0.50 tsp
Pepper, red or cayenne, 0.25 tsp
Salt, 1 tsp
Split Peas, 2 cup
Vegetable Broth, 7.50 cup

What Story Am I in?

However, overfilling your tank has consequences that don't feel loving, like indigestion, lethargy, or feeling bloated, nauseated, headachy, or sleepy. You may feel guilty, regretful, or angry, and judge yourself for lacking willpower when you gain weight and your clothes feel tight.

If you notice your hand reaching toward the cookie jar or the ice cream in the freezer when you're full, walk into another room, away from the food and ask, "What story am I in?" or "What am I believing that's not true?" or "What do I really need right now?" Get quiet and take a few minutes with these questions. Almost always, you will find a painful emotion or some unease lurking underneath this impulse.

Split Pea with Tempeh Meal in a Bowl

Nutritional Info:
Servings Per Recipe: 6
Amount Per Serving
Calories: 246.5
Total Fat: 4.8 g
Cholesterol: 0.0 mg
Sodium: 2,269.0 mg
Total Carbs: 32.7 g
Dietary Fiber: 11.5 g
Protein: 17.5 g

Ingredients:
Pepper, black, 0.50 tsp
Pepper, red or cayenne, 0.25 tsp
Salt, 1 tsp
Split Peas, 2 cup
Vegetable Broth, 7.50 cup
Fakin' Bacon, 9 serving (

The Mosquito Flick

Beliefs that cause you to suffer are big fat lies or, at the very least, partial truths.

Beliefs that cause you to overeat and feel bad only contain a sliver of truth, but that the ego used that sliver to hook you. Thankfully, when you see that you've been suckered—really see it—you become liberated from those beliefs. If they arise again, you can notice them, and flick them away like you would a mosquito.

Turkey Chili/Vegetarian Chili

Preparation Time: 15 minutes

Nutritional Info:
Servings Per Recipe:
6
Amount Per Serving
Calories: 289.9
Total Fat: 6.4 g
Cholesterol: 47.7 mg
Sodium: 1,014.7 mg
Total Carbs: 37.6 g
Dietary Fiber: 9.1 g
Protein: 21.4 g

Nutritional Info:
(Vegetarian)
Servings Per
Recipe: 6
Amount Per Serving
Calories: 280.5
Total Fat: 2.4 g
Cholesterol: 7.7 mg
Sodium: 1,194.3 mg
Total Carbs: 44.7 g
Dietary Fiber: 12 g
Protein: 19.5 g

Ingredients:
Cheddar or Colby Cheese, Low Fat, 1 oz (remove)
Chili powder, 1 tsp
Cumin seed, 2 tsp
Onions, raw, 1 cup, chopped
Baked Potato (baked potatoes), 1 potato (2-1/3" x 4-3/4")
Red Ripe Tomatoes, 5 plum tomato (remove)
Beans, red kidney, 2 cup
Newman's Own Bandito Salsa Mild, 2 Tbsp, 16 tbsp
Trader Joe's Tomato & Roasted Red Pepper Soup,
4 cup
Ground Turkey (lean) 12 ounces or Lightlife Smart
Ground Mexican Style, 2 cup

Directions:
Add all ingredients to a large pot and simmer for ten
minutes. Serve.

Withdraw Your Romantic Projections

Eating is pleasurable, and there's nothing wrong with enjoying food. Yet when food becomes the object of your desire, your secret passion, entertainment, or a naughty indulgence, you've turned it into something it's not—a lover.

Unconsciously, we can imbue food with the power to fill many physical and emotional needs. But it was never designed to do that.

Ultimately, healing means withdrawing our romantic projections, seeing food as nice-tasting nutrition, not the stuff that we can't wait to curl up with and get into our mouths. Rather than, "Oh, sweet brownie, how I love you and long to taste your rich, chocolaty goodness," our food thoughts might sound like, "I'm hungry and it's time to eat. What will I have? My body could use some protein and vegetables. I have X in the house, so I will create Y meal." Although it may not be sexy or exciting, this new way of thinking sets the stage for a healthy, rational, mature relationship with food.

Black Bean Soup

Preparation Time: 15 minutes
Nutritional Info:
Servings Per Recipe: 8
Amount Per Serving
Calories: 154.3
Total Fat: 1.0 g
Cholesterol: 0.7 mg
Sodium: 271.8 mg
Total Carbs: 27.8 g
Dietary Fiber: 8.8 g
Protein: 9.3 g

Ingredients:
Cheddar or Colby Cheese, Low Fat, 1 oz
Chili powder, 2 tbsp
Onions, raw, 0.50 cup, chopped
Beans, black in broth, 4 cup
Imagine Organic Vegetable Broth, 4 cup
Newman's Own Organic Chunky Mild Salsa, one jar.

Directions:
Mash two cans of black beans and broth with a potato
masher or in a blender or food processor. Combine all
ingredients except the onion and cheese in a saucepan
and bring to a boil. Serve topped with cheese and onion
as a garnish.

If You Don't Have Two Minutes
With A Particular Food,
It Really Won't Impact Your Life

If you eat for pleasure, chances are that you see food as your friend, a treat, or a reward rather than just as nourishment. It's a very deeply embedded view in which food becomes larger than life, taking on a glorified and revered position in your life. You blow its importance out of proportion relative to what it can actually offer you. Because you see your relationship with pleasure food as more important to your happiness than it truly is, if you allow yourself to eat it after abstaining from it on a diet, you can easily go hog wild.

The pleasure from eating is fleeting! Soon after you put something in your mouth, the experience of eating is over. That's part of the whole truth that the Child doesn't want you to know.

It's liberating to realize that if you don't have two minutes with a particular food, it really won't impact your life.

Sides

Mustard Greens - Steamed with Garlic, and Miso Sesame Dressing

I use this recipe for preparing any vegetables including kale, collard greens, broccoli, and green beans.

Preparation time: 5 minutes

Nutritional Info:
Servings Per Recipe: 2
Amount Per Serving
Calories: 95.6
Total Fat: 2.4 g
Cholesterol: 0.0 mg
Sodium: 820.3 mg
Total Carbs: 14.7 g
Dietary Fiber: 6.2 g
Protein: 6.2 g

Ingredients:
Garlic, 2 clove
Mustard greens, fresh, 6 cup, chopped
GALEOS miso, 2 tbsp
*Nakano Seasoned Rice Vinegar, 2 tbsp
Soy sauce (tamari), 1 tbsp

Directions:
Wash and chop mustard greens. Steam for one minute. Chop and brown the garlic cloves. Add mustard greens, rice vinegar, tamari and Miso sauce. Heat for one minute. Serve.

Realizing How Untrue Your Thoughts About Food Have Been Means You're Well on Your Way to Thinking about it Differently

When we habitually think about food in a way that creates excitement and pleasurable sensations, it makes food seem wonderfully fun and special, and this can leave us in an emotionally charged trance of sorts. Without realizing it, we slip into another state of consciousness, where seeing the whole truth about food is impossible. Once we realize how untrue and overblown our thinking is about it, we're well on our way to thinking about it differently.

Glorifying food is a habit of believing that we need it to be happy and to feel good. But we don't. As we examine our beliefs about food and discover the truth, we realize that we never needed to get pleasure from food because life itself is pleasurable.

Mashed Butternut Squash with Cinnamon and Nutmeg

Nutritional Info:
Servings Per Recipe: 2
Amount Per Serving
Calories: 87.1
Total Fat: 0.4 g
Cholesterol: 0.0 mg
Sodium: 9.3 mg
Total Carbs: 22.4 g
Dietary Fiber: 6.5 g
Protein: 1.9 g

Ingredients:
Butternut Squash, 2 cup, cubes (buy peeled and chopped)
Nutmeg, ground, .5 tsp
Cinnamon, ground, .5 tsp

Directions:
Bake squash at 350 till soft. Mash and blend with nutmeg and cinnamon

How can I feed my soul and experience the kind of joy that can't fade or turn into its opposite?

With so many other pleasures available, why have so many of us become fixated on and addicted to food? What's its allure? I'd wager that most would say that food captures our hearts and imaginations because it looks, smells, and tastes so good. It activates all five of our senses. From the moment that we lift food-laden forks to our lips, there is no denying the pleasure it gives us. Or is there? Are we totally sure about this pleasure assumption?

Image eating your favorite food all by yourself with no other distractions. Does this sound appealing? If not, why not?

If food were truly the love of your life, why would you need to couple eating with other activities? Why isn't eating, this so-called most pleasurable experience, enough? Hmm? Maybe, just maybe, your idea of eating doesn't match up to the truth about it. Maybe you haven't been seeing the whole truth about food.

There is no denying that while food is in our mouths, it tastes good. Yet prolonging the pleasure means inserting more and more food. And if we do this, we all know what happens. When we follow one bite with another and end up overfilling our stomachs, in no time, the experience of eating shifts into something else. The pleasure turns into pain. The excited anticipation turns into aversion.

The truth about loving food is that it tastes good for only a short while and if we try to draw out its taste pleasure, our love soon turns to hate, and weight gain, guilt, self-castigation, lethargy, and aversion follow in quick succession. Does it really make sense to romanticize an experience when the pleasure you derive from it is so fleeting? Or are there other ways you can take care of yourself that are *truly* fulfilling and nurturing? Ask yourself, "How can I feed my soul and experience the kind of joy that can't fade or turn into its opposite?"

Kale with Rice Vinegar, Garlic, & Tamari

Nutritional Info:
Servings Per Recipe: 2
Amount Per Serving
Calories: 113.1
Total Fat: 1.1 g
Cholesterol: 0.0 mg
Sodium: 1,595.8 mg
Total Carbs: 22.6 g
Dietary Fiber: 5.4 g
Protein: 7.0 g

Ingredients:
Garlic, 2 cloves
Kale, 4 cup, chopped
Soy sauce (tamari), 2 tbsp
rice vinegar, 2 tbsp

Directions:
Wash and chop kale. Steam for one minute. Chop and
brown the garlic cloves. Add the kale, rice vinegar,
and tamari. Heat for one minute. Serve.

What Are Your "9s" and 10s"?

An important part of withdrawing your romanticization of food is finding other activities that are pleasurable and meaningful, other than food. What are other "10's" for you? What do you enjoy that doesn't bring the suffering that accompanies your all-consuming love affair with food? Food may never become a "1" for you, but hopefully, after practicing the Five Steps, you will be able to see it as a "5" or a "6." Today, spend ten or fifteen minutes doing a "9" or a "10."

New Potatoes with Peas and Mint

Nutritional Info:
Servings Per Recipe: 8
Amount Per Serving
Calories: 234.6
Total Fat: 3.8 g
Cholesterol: 0.0 mg
Sodium: 35.5 mg
Total Carbs: 37.6 g
Dietary Fiber: 5.1 g
Protein: 10.6 g

Ingredients:
Peas, fresh, 2 cup
Olive Oil, 2 tbsp
White Wine, 4 fl oz
Fage Greek Yogurt 0% fat, 16 oz
Fresh Chives, 3 tbsp chopped
Mint leaves,8 tbsp chopped
Red Potato, 6 cups parboiled (still firm) chopped

Directions:
Blend all ingredients. Refrigerate and serve cold.

TOILET PAPER

Healing our food issues means that we learn to stop glamorizing food by withdrawing some of our false projections onto it and false meanings we've given to it.

A balanced relationship with food would be more like your relationship with toilet paper. Okay, I admit this is a crude analogy, but with both food and toilet paper, quality is important. They both fill a need (when you need it, you need it!), the experience of using them is quick, and most importantly, there's no need to think about them when you're not using them. It's not like you're going to create an overblown fantasy anticipating the velvety softness of two-ply Cottonelle!

Collard Greens with Ginger Miso Sauce

Nutritional Info
Servings Per Recipe: 2
Amount Per Serving
Calories: 101.5
Total Fat: 7.8 g
Cholesterol: 0.0 mg
Sodium: 531.6 mg
Total Carbs: 6.6 g
Dietary Fiber: 2.7 g
Protein: 3.4 g

Ingredients:
*Genji's Ginger Miso Dressing, 2 tbsp
Collards, 4 cup, chopped
Garlic, 2 cloves
Soy sauce (tamari), 1 tbsp

Directions:
Wash and chop collard greens. Steam for one minute.
Chop and brown the garlic cloves. Add collard greens, rice
vinegar, tamari and Genji's Ginger Miso sauce. Heat for
one minute. Serve.

When You Don't Think About Food, You're Free of it

Take a moment now to notice any romantic thoughts you might have about food and ask if these projections are really true. Can food fulfill you and give you lasting pleasure?

When you go without food and don't think about it, you see the truth: You really don't need food as a source of pleasure. Of course, you need it to survive, but you don't need to have a certain food at a particular time.

When you don't think about food, you're free of it, and you see that you don't need to have a romance with it. Then, your relationship with it can become very practical and healthy.

Instead of dreaming about food like you might fantasize about sex, notice the pleasure in being alive, in performing simple everyday tasks, and in thinking about food in a practical way.

The romantic relationship with food disappears as you see the complete truth about what it can and can't offer you. The way we think about food is the crux of our problems with it. If our romanticism of and longing for food go away, then our problem with food goes away.

Feta Lentil Salad

Nutritional Info:
Servings Per Recipe: 8
Amount Per Serving
Calories: 276.6
Total Fat: 6.0 g
Cholesterol: 5.0 mg
Sodium: 197.1 mg
Total Carbs: 37.1 g
Dietary Fiber: 16.4 g
Protein: 20.0 g

Ingredients:
Olive Oil, 2 tbsp
Lemon Juice, 0.25 cup
Garlic, 2 cloves press
Trader Joes Low Fat Feta, 8 ozs
Beluga Black Lentils, cooked 4 cups

Directions:
Blend all ingredients, refrigerate and serve.

Wild Rice with Cherries and Pistachios

Nutritional Info:
Servings Per Recipe: 4
Amount Per Serving
Calories: 193.2
Total Fat: 7.1 g
Cholesterol: 0.0 mg
Sodium: 748.8 mg
Total Carbs: 27.9 g
Dietary Fiber: 3.0 g
Protein: 5.5 g

Ingredients:
Wild Rice, 1 cup
*pistachios, 0.5 cup
Salt, 1 dash
Vegetable Broth, 3 cup
*Dried Cherries, 0.5 cup

Directions: Bring vegetable stock to a boil. Add wild rice.
Let simmer for 25 minutes. Mix in the cherries, salt and
pistachios. Let sit covered for 5 minutes. If you want the
rice to be less chewy, cook for longer.

Catching Thoughts Before They Sprout into Feelings

Feelings manifest as sensations in the body, making them seem much more real than thoughts. If we feel a certain way, that feeling must be true, right? As if this weren't enough, inflated by self-righteousness, the ego comes up with all the reasons why *we're right* about our feelings, feeding a given emotion with more thoughts, pumping it up until it achieves its desired objective—action. The ego is always looking for a fight, and the worse we feel, the better it likes it.

Feelings come from thoughts. It seems like this should be common knowledge, found in a standard-issue operating manual on how to live as a human being. Just think—if we had known that feelings come from thoughts when we were children, we could have learned to deal with our stressful thoughts by either ignoring or questioning them. In fact, we could have avoided creating negative feelings in the first place!

Quick, Easy Meals Made with Prepared Sauces

Thai Green Curry Chicken with Vegetables and Brown Rice

Nutritional Info:
Servings Per Recipe: 4
Amount Per Serving
Calories: 290.3
Total Fat: 7.2 g
Cholesterol: 68.4 mg
Sodium: 813.1 mg
Total Carbs: 39.1 g
Dietary Fiber: 5.0 g
Protein: 32.7 g

Ingredients:
Chicken Breast, no skin, 2 breast, bone and skin removed, sliced into one inch strips
Onions, raw, 1 cup, chopped
brown rice (1 cup cooked), 2 serving
Snow Peas, fresh, 1 cup
Best Choice Broccoli Florets, 1 cup
Thai Green Curry, 1.5 cup
Carrots, raw, 1 cup, chopped
Basil, 4 tbsp
Bean sprouts, 1 cup

Directions:
Spray a large nonstick skillet with cooking spray. Brown the chicken on both sides about 4 minutes per side using medium high heat. Add all of the vegetables, stirring constantly. Add the curry sauce and cover. Heat the brown rice in the microwave for 2 minutes. Serve by placing the rice on a plate covering it with the chicken, sauce and vegetables.

Staying in Alignment with Essence

Maintaining our emotional hygiene by debunking negative thoughts can become second nature—the only sane way to live.

We have the power to stop creating negative emotions. When a stressful belief arises, we can catch it and say to ourselves, "Oh, that's just conditioning." and ignore it.

If we buy into a belief and accidentally created a negative feeling, we can ask, "What am I believing right now that's causing me to feel this way?" That question can yank us out of the ego and transport us back to the rational, pleasant world of the true self.

Chicken with Vodka Sauce

Nutritional Info:
Servings Per Recipe: 4
Amount Per Serving
Calories: 310.9
Total Fat: 5.0 g
Cholesterol: 68.4 mg
Sodium: 301.0 mg
Total Carbs: 31.9 g
Dietary Fiber: 3.6 g
Protein: 33.0 g

Ingredients:
Newman's Own Vodka Sauce, 1/2 cup, 1 cup
Chicken Breast, no skin, 2 breast, bone and skin removed
Green Beans (snap), 2 cup
brown rice (1 cup cooked), 2 serving

Directions:
Spray a large nonstick skillet with cooking spray. Brown the chicken on both sides about 6 minutes per side using medium high heat. While the chicken is cooking, steam the green beans for 3 minutes and heat the brown rice in the microwave for 2 minutes. Pour the vodka sauce over the chicken. Cover the skillet for 30 seconds. Serve by placing the rice on a plate covering it with the chicken and sauce and putting the collards on the side.

You Are that which Is Aware of Emotion

We have become accustomed to listening to and believing stressful thoughts that create anger, sadness, and fear. With practice, though, we can learn to catch feelings before they form. We can form a new habit of ignoring the egoic mind and seeing thoughts as simply results of our conditioning.

One reason our feelings feel so real and overwhelming is that we identify or merge with them. We become the anger or sadness or fear. We think that it's *our* anger and feel self-righteous about it: "It's mine, and I have a right to express it, and you'd better respect it!"

But who says that feelings belong to us? Or even that thoughts belong to us? Both arise and subside unbidden.

If we feel ownership of our emotions and believe they're meaningful, it will be harder to let them arise and subside naturally. We'll want to hold on to them, feel their power, and feed them with more thoughts and beliefs that justify their presence. Then, we'll want others to validate our position and our right to feel what we feel. If you remember that you are *that which is aware* of emotion, rather than the emotion itself, it will have far less power over you. From this vantage point, you can watch the action without getting involved in it. For example, anger happens. It arises, it's felt, it does its dance, it subsides—and you remain unchanged. You are only the space in which anger arises and are completely unsullied by it.

Chicken or Meatless Ball Korma with Broccoli and Brown Rice

Nutritional
Info
Servings Per Recipe: 4
Amount Per Serving
Calories: 366.3
Total Fat: 8.7 g
Cholesterol: 77.3 mg
Sodium: 515.5 mg
Total Carbs: 36.3 g
Dietary Fiber: 5.5 g
Protein: 32.3 g

Ingredients:
Chicken Breast, no skin, 2 breast, bone and skin removed
brown rice (1 cup cooked), 2 servings, frozen from Trader Joes
Best Choice Broccoli Florets, 4 cup
Trader Joes Korma Simmer Sauce, 1.17 cup

Directions:
Spray a large nonstick skillet with cooking spray. Brown the chicken on both sides about 6 minutes per side using medium high heat. While the chicken is cooking, steam the broccoli for 3 minutes and heat the brown rice in the microwave for 2 minutes. Pour the Korma sauce over the chicken. Cover the skillet for 30 seconds. Serve by placing the rice on a plate covering it with the chicken and sauce and putting the collards on the side.

Shoulding

Whenever we're upset about what's happening, we're arguing with reality. Life in the form of a particular situation has already happened. It's a fact, and there's nothing we can do about it. As author Byron Katie says, "When we fight with life we lose, but only 100% of the time!" Our resistance to life is created by the thought "This shouldn't be happening." This is the most common way that we cause our own suffering.

Whenever we're irritated by a situation—we're waiting in a traffic jam or someone breaks a promise—the mind tends to jump in and proclaim that this or that *should* be different: "There *should* be more staff on the cash registers so that people don't have to wait for such a long time." "They *shouldn't* make a promise they can't keep." "They *should* have known better." "This slow car in front of me *should* go faster."

Notice what happens when you use the word "should." There's an immediate contraction in your body. You're resisting life and that doesn't feel good. Your perspective narrows down to a tiny sliver of the truth about a situation and you miss seeing the whole picture. Seeing only the reasons why things *should* be different, you don't consider the possible benefits of the situation.

Salmon or Tofu Rogan Josh with Collard Greens and Brown Rice

Nutritional Info
Servings Per Recipe: 4
Amount Per Serving
Calories: 332.1
Total Fat: 12.4 g
Cholesterol: 80.5 mg
Sodium: 671.7 mg
Total Carbs: 36.5 g
Dietary Fiber: 4.0 g
Protein: 33.5 g

Nutritional Info
Servings Per Recipe: 4
Amount Per Serving
Calories: 199.8
Total Fat: 4.8 g
Cholesterol: 0.0 mg
Sodium: 778.2 mg
Total Carbs: 38.7 g
Dietary Fiber: 4.0 g
Protein: 17.2 g

Atlantic Salmon (fish), 16 oz
Truly Indian Rogan Josh, 16 oz
Collards, 4 cup, chopped
brown rice (1 cup cooked), 2 servings, frozen from Trader Joes

Directions:
Spray a large nonstick skillet with cooking spray. Brown the salmon on both sides about 3 minutes per side using medium high heat. While the salmon is cooking, steam the collard greens for 2 minutes and heat the brown rice in the microwave for 2 minutes Pour the Rogan Josh our over the salmon. Cover the skillet for 30 seconds. Serve by placing the rice on a plate covering it with the salmon and sauce and putting the collards on the side.

Letting it be Okay to be in Reaction

Today, if you're standing in a long checkout line at the supermarket or stuck in traffic, consider the possibility that waiting provides an opportunity for quiet contemplation.

If someone lets you down or breaks a promise, it gives you a chance to learn tolerance or discernment: Remember how it felt when you made a promise that you didn't keep or let someone down, and sidestep judgment and learn compassion and forgiveness, instead.

Today if something happens that you don't like, look at the potential benefit that comes with this new development. You don't have to jump right to the downside or what you think should be happening, as you might have done in the past. Considering the benefit eliminates the reaction altogether. Don't be discouraged if it takes a lot of practice to get to this point.

If you notice anger arising today, you can recognize that your conditioning is coming up in the form of anger and say, "Oh, that's just my conditioning." This noticing helps you dis-identify with your negative story and let it go. If you're quick enough, you'll notice and dis-identify with it before the anger or stress has a chance to erupt in your body!

If you get triggered today, acknowledge it. You can say something like, "Wow, I've really been triggered," or "I'm really in reaction." Noticing and telling yourself the truth brings you back to the present moment, takes you out of the story you're running and into the Wise Witness. *Be gentle with yourself and let it be okay that you're in reaction.* Ironically, this will move you into acceptance! Once you're in acceptance, even if you found it by accepting the fact that you're in resistance, you can go back to your true self!

Tex Mex Pita Sandwich

Nutritional Info:
Servings Per Recipe: 4
Amount Per Serving
Calories: 369.8
Total Fat: 16.9 g
Cholesterol: 0.0 mg
Sodium: 662.6 mg
Total Carbs: 43.0 g
Dietary Fiber: 10.5 g
Protein: 18.7 g

Ingredients:
Amy's Kitchen Texas Veggie Burgers, 4, lightly browned
*Avocado (Medium), 1, remove fruit from the skin and slice
Bread, pita, whole-wheat, 2 pita, large (6-1/2" dia) sliced in half.
Romaine Lettuce, 0.5 cup, shredded
Red Ripe Tomatoes, 2 plum tomatoes sliced
Onions, raw, 1 small sliced thinly
*Humus, Sabra Chipotle, 4 servings

Directions:
Spread humus in each pita half. Place a burger in each half and then add one quarter of the avocado, lettuce, tomato, and onion. Brown pita halves on both sides in a skillet.

Not Now Maybe Later

When we're bored, we tell ourselves the unhappy story that whatever is happening is uninteresting and not what we were hoping for from life. We feel restless and dissatisfied. Oftentimes, when we tell ourselves a story that results in boredom, we move into default mode—reaching for something tasty. We allow the Child to take over, and see food solely as a source of pleasure. One way to avoid reaching for food when boredom strikes is to say to the Child, just as we might to a persistent two-year-old, "Not now—maybe later."

Tempeh Rueben Sandwich

Nutritional Info:
Servings Per Recipe: 4
Amount Per Serving
Calories: 309.6
Fat: 9.3 g
Cholesterol: 14.1 mg
Sodium: 1,729.6 mg
Total Carbs: 35.6 g
Dietary Fiber: 7.5 g
Protein: 21.6 g

Ingredients:
Bread, pita, whole-wheat, 2 pita, large cut in half (6-1/2" dia)
*Sauerkraut, 1 cup
*Kroger Fat Free Swiss Cheese Slices, 8 servings
Thousand Island Salad Dressing, 4 tbsp
Fakin' Bacon, cut package in half, brown strips

Directions:
Spread salad dressing in each pita half. Add one quarter of the cheese, sauerkraut, and Fakin Bacon. Brown pita halves on both sides in a skillet, until the cheese melts.

See the Whole Truth of Food When You're Bored

When we're bored, we tell ourselves the unhappy story that whatever is happening is uninteresting and not what we were hoping for from life. We feel restless and dissatisfied. Oftentimes, when we tell ourselves a story that results in boredom, we move into default mode—reaching for something tasty. We allow the Child to take over, and see food solely as a source of pleasure. One way to avoid reaching for food when boredom strikes is to say to the Child, just as we might to a persistent two-year-old, "Not now—maybe later."

The Wise Witness remembers the whole truth about pleasure food, that even though it may taste nice for a few fleeting seconds, it can't alleviate boredom. If we eat it and we're not hungry, it may not taste as good as we had imagined or we may overeat it and end up feeling worse because we gave into our craving. Seeing the whole truth about food from the perspective of the Wise Witness, interrupts the automatic tendency to reach for food when we're bored.

Healthy Falafel Sandwich

Nutritional Info:
Servings Per Recipe: 4
Amount Per Serving
Calories: 367.8
Total Fat: 18.6 g
Cholesterol: 5.0 mg
Sodium: 598.6 mg
Total Carbs: 34.1 g
Dietary Fiber: 6.9 g
Protein: 21.8 g

Ingredients:
Bread, pita, whole-wheat, 2 pita, large (6-1/2" dia)
Romaine Lettuce (salad), 0.5 cup, shredded
Onion raw, 1 small, sliced thin
tomatoes sliced thin.
*Tahini, 8 tbsp
Quorn Meatless Balls, 4 servings,(16 meatballs) thawed
and browned

Directions:
Cut the pita pockets in half. Stuff each pita half with
one quarter of the lettuce, tomatoes, onions, and
meatballs. Holding the pita open, drizzle with tahini
sauce. Serve.

Allow Feelings to Be Present

At their core, fear and worry are about survival. The egoic mind invents a scary future and you're instantly trapped in fear's clutches. 90% of the things you fear will never happen.

Just because fear and worry arise doesn't mean you have to avoid them through food. They can't hurt you and like all other feelings, they eventually dissipate. You can allow them to be present and learn to tolerate them after all. The best way to deal with fear and worry is to ask, "What's the worst thing that could happen?" Then you see that even if the worst thing happens, you can deal with it and then, fear lets go of you and you can rest.

Chili Baked Potatoes

Nutritional Info:
Servings Per Recipe: 1
Amount Per Serving
Calories: 194.1
Total Fat: 2.1 g
Cholesterol: 6.0 mg
Sodium: 181.3 mg
Total Carbs: 34.2 g
Dietary Fiber: 2.3 g
Protein: 10.0 g

Ingredients:
Cheddar or Colby Cheese, Low Fat, 1 oz
Baked Potato (baked potatoes), 1 potato (2-1/3" x 4-3/4")
1/6 of a recipe of vegetarian chili

Directions:
Wash the potato. Poke holes throughout with a fork. Bake the potato for one hour at 350 degrees. Open the potato by slicing ¾ of the way through in a cross formation. Mash interior. Open and pour in one serving of vegetarian chili.

Slow Down the Action.

One important step in dealing with feelings is to *slow down the action*.

Addictive patterns make us go into zombie mode, distracting us and keeping us from being present in the moment. Set the intention and ask for help from the Wise Witness to *be present* when an eating compulsion strikes. By setting this intention, you commit to your own healing and plant your feet squarely on Recovery Road. It's as if you're saying, "I'm ready to move on and transform my dysfunctional relationship with food."

After you've set the intention to be present, even if you continue to go unconscious the next 20, 50, or 500 times the impulse to eat comes up, something in you will remember that intention, and eventually you'll be able to interrupt the emotional food-stuffing response. The more often you can interrupt your usual pattern, the easier it will become. Just as you created the old habit of eating in response to frightening and uncomfortable emotions, you can create a new habit of awareness by slowing down the action and removing yourself from the danger zone—wherever the food is.

Spaghetti Squash with Marinara Sauce and Turkey Meatballs (Quorn Meatless Balls)

Nutritional Info
Servings Per Recipe: 4
Amount Per Serving
Calories: 374.9
Total Fat: 18.4 g
Cholesterol: 62.4 mg
Sodium: 1,117.6 mg
Total Carbs: 29.7 g
Dietary Fiber: 6.5 g
Protein: 26.9 g

Nutritional Info
(vegetarian)
Servings Per Recipe: 4
Amount Per Serving
Calories: 382.1
Total Fat: 15.8 g
Cholesterol: 27.4 mg
Sodium: 1,464.4 mg
Total Carbs: 36.0 g
Dietary Fiber: 7.2 g
Protein: 28.7 g

Ingredients:
Parmesan Cheese, grated, 4 oz
Pepper, black, 0.25 tsp
Olive Oil, 1 tbsp
Black Olives, chopped 10 jumbo
Garlic, 4 cloves (remove)
Onions, raw, 2 cup, chopped
Spaghetti Squash, 4 cups
Tomato Sauce, 1 cup
Red Ripe Tomatoes, 6 Italian tomato
Turkey, Ground turkey, 93% lean, 8 oz
Basil, ground 1 tsp
Oregano, ground, 1 tsp
Parsley, 1 tbsp
Bay leaf, 1

Directions:
Bake squash for an hour. While squash is baking, sauté garlic and onions in olive oil in a saucepan using medium heat until soft. Blend in the all other ingredients, except the parmesan cheese and cook over medium heat, stirring frequently. Set aside. Scoop cooked squash onto a serving platter. Top with sauce. Sprinkle with cheese and serve.

What Story Am I In?

We've come to believe that when the Child comes on the scene, we have no choice but to listen and follow her directions. The truth, though, is that the past is *not* a reliable predictor of the future. Just because you've reached for food 620,000 times before doesn't mean you have to do it now. You can choose health over your conditioning, your true self over the ego.

Rather than listening to the Child coaxing you down a self-destructive road to food hell, ask yourself if you're willing to try something different. Just this once, are you willing to stop the action and not reach for food?

Instead of stuffing down the depression or sadness with food, could you allow it to be present and ask yourself, "What story am I in right now? What am I believing that's causing me to feel flattened and down on myself and life?" You can even tell the Child that she can still eat later, if that's what she wants, but not right now. The next time depression or sadness is on the scene, try this experiment and see what happens.

Veggie Quesadillas

Nutritional Info
Servings Per Recipe: 4
Amount Per Serving
Calories: 180.4
Total Fat: 7.3 g
Cholesterol: 15.0 mg
Sodium: 316.5 mg
Total Carbs: 11.8 g
Dietary Fiber: 4.7 g
Protein: 14.7 g

Ingredients:
Trader Joes Low Carb Whole Wheat Tortillas, 4 serving
Trader Joe's Shredded Lite Mexican Blend Cheese, 1 cup
Onions, raw, 2 cup, chopped
Mushrooms, fresh, 2 cup, pieces or slices
Garlic, 3 cloves
Salt, 1 dash
Pepper, black, 1 dash
Zucchini, 1 cup, sliced
Spinach, fresh, 1 cup
Cooking Spray

Directions:
Coat a large skillet with cooking spray and sauté the vegetables and the salt and pepper till soft. Remove from the pan. Recoat that pan with cooking spray and warm the tortillas over medium heat. Sprinkle one quarter of the cheese over one half of each tortilla, add one quarter of the vegetables and close the tortilla to create a half moon shape. Brown on both sides and serve while warm.

How Boredom Is Experienced From the True Self

If you eat to numb out, you miss the opportunity to heal whatever conditioning is arising.

The next time you're bored, ask yourself "What is my true self's experience of boredom?" You know the ego's experience, but become aware of how your true self *just notices* the boredom. It isn't the generator of the feeling (the ego is), and it isn't affected by it either. It just notices boredom arising and doesn't evaluate it as something to like or not like. It isn't trying to get life to conform to a certain feeling. It's just humming along, okay with everything as it is.

When boredom arises, you can become aware of it and realize that it's not who you really are. In other words, you can dis-identify with it. Who you are is able to notice the ego being bored. Simply allow the feeling of boredom to be present and reengage in what you're doing. When you allow a negative feeling to be present without trying to make it to dissipate or when you're fully engaged in what you're doing, you're not thinking. And if you're not thinking, you automatically align with your true self and you can't be bored. What a blessing!

Tacos

Nutritional Info:
Servings Per Recipe: 4
Amount Per Serving
Calories: 326.7
Total Fat: 9.2 g
Cholesterol: 63.5 mg
Sodium: 757.7 mg
Total Carbs: 37.8 g
Dietary Fiber: 7.0 g
Protein: 26.4 g

Nutritional Info:
(vegetarian)
Servings Per Recipe: 4
Amount Per Serving
Calories: 259.2
Total Fat: 3.1 g
Cholesterol: 3.5 mg
Sodium: 635.6 mg
Total Carbs: 40.8 g
Dietary Fiber: 9.0 g
Protein: 18.2 g

Ingredients:
Pam spray
Ground Turkey (93% lean) or Lightlife Smart Ground-
Mexican Style, browned, 4 servings
Salsa, 2 cups
Romaine Lettuce (salad), 2 cups, shredded
Red Ripe Tomatoes, 1 cup, chopped or sliced
Onions, raw, 1 cup, chopped
Cheddar or Colby Cheese, Low Fat, .5 cup, diced
Corn Tortillas, 8 tortilla, medium (approx. 6" dia)

Directions: Cover a large skillet with a coat of cooking
spray. Using medium heat place for tortillas in the pan,
folding each in half (but not to the breaking point.) Heat on
each side. When the tortillas hold their shape, remover
them from the pan and fill them with Turkey or Smart
Ground, lettuce, tomatoes, onions and cheese. Top with
salsa and serve immediately.

The Cycle of a Craving

When a craving is on the scene, it can feel like it's driving and we're just along for the ride. When we finally fulfill our desire, finally bite into that donut or piece of chocolate cake, we *credit the food* for the momentary bliss we feel. But we have it backwards. *It's the craving that caused the suffering*, not our being deprived of the object of our desire. And *it's the elimination of the craving that caused the bliss,* not the food. We feel great because we're no longer burdened by the craving, yet we mistakenly give the credit to the chocolate cake.

If we overeat the chocolate cake, the suffering isn't really gone, but transformed into the guilt and self-loathing we feel after indulging. The ego keeps our thinking compartmentalized so that in the throes of a craving, we think only about the object of our desire, not the complete experience. We become the Scarlett O'Haras of eating, opining, "I'll think about that tomorrow." This is how we dupe ourselves into indulging and suffering again and again. We think only about the fleeting pleasure we get from fulfilling the craving and ignore the negative repercussions.

Vegetarian Tostadas

Nutritional Info:
Servings Per Recipe: 4
Amount Per Serving
Calories: 338.5
Total Fat: 2.8 g
Cholesterol: 3.5 mg
Sodium: 641.0 mg
Total Carbs: 51.4 g
Dietary Fiber: 14.9 g
Protein: 28.1 g

Ingredients:
Cheddar or Colby Cheese, Low Fat, 0.50 cup, diced
Salsa, 1 cup
Romaine Lettuce (salad), 2 cup, shredded
Onions, raw, 1 cup, chopped
Red Ripe Tomatoes, 1 cup, chopped or sliced
Beans, black, 2 cup
Corn Tortillas, 4 tortilla, medium (approx. 6" dia)
Lightlife Smart Ground Mexican Style, 1.33 cup
Fage Greek Yogurt 0% fat, 6 oz

Directions:
Heat the corn tortillas in a skillet on both sides, until crisp. Place
tortillas on serving places. Spread black beans over the surface, add
the Lightlife Smart Ground, lettuce, tomatoes, onions, and cheese.
Add a dollop of salsa and yogurt, then serve.

Telling Yourself the Truth about a Food You're Addicted to

When a craving hits we fool ourselves when we tell ourselves that we can just have a little of what we desire and then stop. But if we're addicted to a food, it's very difficult to stick to that plan. Most of us end up overeating because we don't find the satisfaction we expect, and there's no clear signal to stop other than the pain of an overstuffed belly.

Skinny Thinking is about telling yourself the truth. If you could eat just a little of something you crave, you wouldn't suffer the physical, emotional, and spiritual consequences that often go hand in hand with addictive pleasures. You would break the cycle and take your power back. Unfortunately, most people with food issues can't do this.

When you hear that familiar voice inside your head demanding "I want to eat this now," you can be sure the Child is on the scene. The wise adult part of us wants to eat a particular food because it's part of our nutritional agenda for the day.

The Child gets us into trouble, and the more we can recognize her, the less power she has over us. Every time you decide not to respond to the child, you reduce its power. The more you can recognize the Child aspect of yourself, the easier it will be to align with the Wise Witness and take your power back.

Turkey Tostadas

Nutritional Info:
Servings Per Recipe: 4
Amount Per Serving
Calories: 370.1
Total Fat: 7.9 g
Cholesterol: 53.5 mg
Sodium: 517.8 mg
Total Carbs: 44.7 g
Dietary Fiber: 12.1 g
Protein: 32.8 g

Ingredients:
Cheddar or Colby Cheese, Low Fat, 0.50 cup, diced
Salsa, 1 cup
Romaine Lettuce (salad), 2 cup, shredded
Onions, raw, 1 cup, chopped
Red Ripe Tomatoes, 1 cup, chopped or sliced
Beans, black, 2 cup
Corn Tortillas, 4 tortilla, medium (approx. 6" dia)
Fage Greek Yogurt 0% fat, 6 oz
Salt, 1 dash
Pepper, black, 1 dash
Chili powder, 1 tsp
*Turkey, Ground turkey, 93% lean, 10 oz (brown in a skillet)

Directions:
Heat the corn tortillas in a skillet on both sides, until crisp. Place tortillas on serving places. Spread black beans over the surface, add the turkey, lettuce, tomatoes, onions, and cheese. Add a dollop of salsa and yogurt, then serve.

The Ego's Version of Following a Craving Versus the Actual Experience

The Ego's Version: *Craving → Obtaining the Object of Desire → Fulfillment*

The Complete Experience: *Craving → Indulgence → Momentary Pleasure Due to Elimination of the Desire → Guilt, Self-Loathing, and Weight Gain*

Chicken Teriyaki

Nutritional Info:
Servings Per Recipe: 4
Amount Per Serving
Calories: 201.0
Total Fat: 1.6 g
Cholesterol: 68.5 mg
Sodium: 1,086.6 mg
Total Carbs: 10.7 g
Dietary Fiber: 0.3 g
Protein: 29.6 g

Ingredients:
Apple juice, unsweetened, 0.25 cup
Garlic, 2 cloves
Ginger Root, 3 tsp
Water, tap, 1 cup (8 fl oz)
Soy sauce (tamari), 4 tbsp
Cornstarch, 0.13 cup
Chicken Breast, no skin, 2 breast, bone and skin removed
White Wine, 4 fl oz
Orange Juice, .5 cup
Cooking Spray

Directions:
Spray a large nonstick skillet with cooking spray. Brown the
chicken breasts on both sides about 6 minutes per side using
medium high heat. Whisk together the teriyaki sauce, white wine
and orange juice and pour over the chicken. Cover the skillet,
reduce heat to low, and simmer until chicken is no longer pink in
the middle (about 10-15 minutes), turning the chicken several
times as it cooks. Serve.

Teriyaki Sauce

Nutritional Info:
Servings Per Recipe: 4
Amount Per Serving
Calories: 37.4
Total Fat: 0.1 g
Cholesterol: 0.0 mg
Sodium: 1,008.0 mg
Total Carbs: 7.4 g
Dietary Fiber: 0.3 g
Protein: 2.0 g

Ingredients:
Apple juice, unsweetened, 0.25 cup
Garlic, 2 cloves (remove)
Ginger Root, 3 tsp
Water, tap, 1 cup (8 fl oz)
Soy sauce (tamari), 4 tbsp
Cornstarch, 0.13 cup

Directions:
In your saucepan stir constantly while adding 1 c of water, brown
sugar, soy sauce, ginger, garlic and bring to a boil. Take the
cornstarch and dissolve it in the apple juice and add to the sauce.
Consistently stirring allows the sauce to thicken. If your not happy
with the thickness of the sauce then add more water or soy sauce.

Two Sides of the Desire Coin

Slow down and notice what happens during a meal. When you first sit down, assuming you're hungry, the first few bites taste delicious. But as you move toward satiation, the experience changes, the law of diminishing returns sets in, and each successive bite becomes less pleasurable. Once you're satiated, the pleasure drops off even faster, until each additional bite becomes downright unpleasant!

Eating pleasure food has a tendency to turn into overeating pleasure food. One of the characteristics of pleasure food is that it tastes so darn good that it's hard to stop eating it. How can you be expected to resist eating more of something that was designed to be irresistible? Even when you're stuffed and your stomach is groaning, you still want to taste more. We delude ourselves into thinking that if we continue eating, we can squeeze a bit more pleasure out of the experience, but alas, all we get is pain.

The human impulse to hold on to pleasure and avoid pain is an important part of the whole picture of food. But we live in a world where desire is governed by duality, and overindulging in pleasure is inexorably linked to pain. Just like trying to separate two sides of a coin, you can't peel the pleasure away from the pain.

Spaghetti Squash with Raw Tomatoes, Fresh Basil, Garlic, and Brie

Nutritional Info:
Servings Per Recipe: 5
Amount Per Serving
Calories: 294.9
Total Fat: 18.9 g
Cholesterol: 24.0 mg
Sodium: 652.5 mg
Total Carbs: 22.1 g
Dietary Fiber: 4.6 g
Protein: 13.7 g

Ingredients:
Pepper, black, 1 tsp
Basil, 40 leaves
Salt, 0.50 tsp
Garlic, 3 cloves
Spaghetti Squash, 8 cup
Red Ripe Tomatoes, 6 plum tomato
Lite Brie Trader Joes, 8 serving
Olive Oil, .25 cup

Directions:
Bake a large spaghetti squash at 375 degrees for one hour. While the squash is cooking blend the rest of the ingredients. When the squash is fully baked, slice in half, and remove the meat of the squash. Blend the squash with the rest of the ingredients and serve. You may also chill it and serve.

A Pragmatic Relationship with Food

Food tantalizes our senses, beckoning us with mouthwatering aromas and titillating tastes and textures. Compounded by the fact that, as human beings, we're programmed to love food, we have a perfect storm for an overeating and weight-control disaster. Eating is pleasurable, and there's nothing wrong with enjoying food. Yet when food becomes the object of our desires, our secret passion, entertainment, or a naughty indulgence, we've turned it into something it's not—a lover.

Unconsciously, we can imbue food with the power to fill many physical and emotional needs. It becomes our ideal friend and lover who is always available, never lets us down, never puts us down, and never says no. Epitomizing fidelity, no matter what is happening in our lives, whether we feel on top of the world or down in the dumps, food is there to keep us company. For the fleeting moment it spends in our mouth, our favorite food always delivers.

Ultimately, healing means withdrawing our romantic projections, seeing food as nice-tasting nutrition, not the stuff that we can't wait to curl up with and get into our mouths. Rather than, "Oh, sweet brownie, how I love you and long to taste your rich, chocolaty goodness," our food thoughts might sound like, "I'm hungry and it's time to eat. What will I have? My body could use some protein and vegetables. I have X in the house, so I will create Y meal." Although it may not be sexy or exciting, this new way of thinking sets the stage for a healthy, rational, mature relationship with food.

Chicken with Vodka Sauce

Nutritional Info:
Servings Per Recipe: 4
Amount Per Serving
Calories: 310.9
Total Fat: 5.0 g
Cholesterol: 68.4 mg
Sodium: 301.0 mg
Total Carbs: 31.9 g
Dietary Fiber: 3.6 g
Protein: 33.0 g

Ingredients:
Newman's Own Vodka Sauce, 1/2 cup, 1 cup
Chicken Breast, no skin, 2 breast, bone and skin removed
Green Beans (snap), 2 cup (steamed)
Brown rice (1 cup cooked), 2 serving (frozen from Trader Joes)
Cooking Spray

Directions:
Coat a skillet with cooking spray and Brown the chicken breast on both sides using medium heat. Add Vodka Sauce. Place green beans in a steamer. Steam for 5 minutes or until tender. Heat brown rice in the microwave for 2 minutes. Scoop rice onto serving plate cover with a chicken breast and sauce. Place green beans on the side. Serve.

Desserts

Carob (Chocolate)Banana Brownies

Preparation time:
10 minutes

Baking Time:
20-30 minutes

Nutritional Info:
Servings Per Recipe: 8
Amount Per Serving
Calories: 199.9
Total Fat: 4.0 g
Cholesterol: 93.8 mg
Sodium: 306.7 mg
Total Carbs: 45.4 g
Dietary Fiber: 5.4 g
Protein: 4.2 g

Ingredients:
Banana, fresh, 4 large (8" to 8-7/8" long) mashed
Pure Vanilla Extract 1 T
Salt, 1 t
Butter, salted, melted, 1 T
oat flour, 2 cups
carob powder, 1 cup or 4 squares of unsweetened baking chocolate
3 eggs beaten

Directions:
Blend all ingredients. Pour into a Pyrex baking pan that has been
sprayed with cooking spray. Bake at 325 degrees for 20-25 minutes.
Bake for longer if you prefer firmer brownies. Cool and serve.

Pleasure

If you eat for pleasure, chances are that you see food as your friend, a treat, or a reward rather than just as nourishment. It's a very deeply embedded view in which food becomes larger than life, taking on a glorified and revered position in your life. You blow its importance out of proportion relative to what it can actually offer you. Because you see your relationship with pleasure food as more important to your happiness than it truly is, if you allow yourself to eat it after abstaining from it on a diet, you can easily go hog wild.

But it's important to notice that the pleasure from eating is fleeting! Soon after you put something in your mouth, the experience of eating is over. That's part of the whole truth that the Child doesn't want you to know. It can be liberating to realize that if you don't have two minutes with a particular food, it really won't impact your life.

When we habitually think about food in a way that creates excitement and pleasurable sensations, it makes food seem wonderfully fun and special, and this can leave us in an emotionally charged trance of sorts. Without realizing it, we slip into another state of consciousness, where seeing the whole truth about food is impossible. Once we realize how untrue and overblown our thinking is about it, we're well on our way to thinking about it differently.

Glorifying food is a habit of believing that we need it to be happy and to feel good. But we don't. As we examine our beliefs about food and discover the truth, we realize that we never needed to get pleasure from food because life itself is pleasurable.

Raspberry Brownies

Preparation time:
10 minutes

Baking Time:
20-30 minutes

Nutritional Info
Servings Per Recipe: 8
Amount Per Serving
Calories: 207.6
Total Fat: 4.1 g
Cholesterol: 93.8 mg
Sodium: 306.8 mg
Total Carbs: 47.2 g
Dietary Fiber: 6.4 g
Protein: 4.3 g

Ingredients:
Banana, fresh, 4 large (8" to 8-7/8" long) mashed
Pure Vanilla Extract 1 T
Salt, 1 t
Butter, salted, melted, 1 T
oat flour, 2 cups
carob powder, 1 cup or 4 squares of unsweetened baking chocolate
3 eggs beaten

Directions:
Blend all ingredients. Pour into a Pyrex baking pan that has been
sprayed with cooking spray. Bake at 325 degrees for 20-25 minutes.
Bake for longer if you prefer firmer brownies. Cool and serve.

The Child

When you hear that familiar voice inside your head demanding "I want to eat this now," you can be sure the Child is on the scene. On the other hand, the wise adult part of us wants to eat a particular food because it's part of our nutritional agenda for the day. The Child gets us into trouble, and the more we can recognize her, the less power she has over us. Every time we decide not to respond to her, we reduce her power.

If we're very identified with the Child, however, it can feel like we have no choice with regard to her demands. They can feel like life or death imperatives. "Eat this now, not two minutes from now," she says. "I want it now. Let me have it. I'll hate you if you don't give it to me."

The Child rationalizes, plays games, and hooks us with partial truths about food that have nothing to do with its nutrition (the real reason we eat it), focusing on pleasure, not what the body actually needs. Unconcerned about what's good or bad for her, she just wants what she wants and doesn't see the consequences of fulfilling her desires in the way an adult would.

The more you can recognize the Child aspect of yourself, the easier it will be to align with the Wise Witness and take your power back. The Wise Witness knows there's a price to pay for following this pleasure-seeking principle, and if you strengthen your Wise Witness by listening to it more, you will feel less compelled to follow the dictates of the Child.

Cream Cheese Brownies

Preparation time:
20 minutes

Baking Time:
20-30 minutes

Nutritional Info
Servings Per Recipe: 8
Amount Per Serving
Calories: 236.2
Total Fat: 4.3 g
Cholesterol: 100.9 mg
Sodium: 334.9 mg
Total Carbs: 52.5 g
Dietary Fiber: 6.1 g
Protein: 5.8 g

Ingredients:

Brownie base:
Banana, fresh, 4 large (8" to 8-7/8" long) mashed
Pure Vanilla Extract 1 T
Salt, 1 t
Butter, salted, melted, 1 T
oat flour, 2 cups
carob powder, 1 cup or 4 squares of unsweetened baking chocolate
3 eggs beaten

Cream Cheese Topping:
Fage Greek Yogurt 0% fat, 4 oz
Banana, fresh, 1 cup, mashed
oat flour, .75 serving
Vanilla Extract, 1 tsp
Salt, .125 tsp

Directions:
Blend all ingredients. Pour into a pry baking pan that has been sprayed with cooking spray. Bake at 325 degrees for 20-25 minutes. Bake for longer if you prefer firmer brownies. Cool and serve.

Learning Not to Follow the Child

When the desire to eat pleasure food arises, just recognize it: "Oh, that's the Child." Doing this lessens the Child's power because, all of a sudden, you realize that what you thought you wanted is really just what the Child wants. In seeing this, you've dis-identified with the Child. When you see the truth, it interrupts the pattern and cuts through it.

The two benefits of dis-identifying with the Child are that it weakens the ego and leaves you with time to make a more rational choice. Instead of indulging, you might say, "I'm not going to indulge the Child right now." Or, like a wise parent, you might just say "no" to it: "No, you can't have another cookie." Or, from a place of choice and detachment, you might decide, "Okay, let's have some pleasure." In that case, you're choosing rather than reacting based on compulsion.

When you react out of habit, it feels like you have no choice. But when you're aligned with the Wise Witness, you're free to make a choice. When you're listening to and obeying the Child, you're bound. That's a huge difference! The goal is to recognize that you're not the Child and develop enough distance from her so that you're free from unconsciously acquiescing to her and indulging her demands. When you see that the "I" that craves is the ego and *not you*, it is much easier to ignore a craving. You become *that which is noticing the Child craving food.* From that place of dis-identification, you can turn your attention elsewhere. Don't be discouraged if, in the beginning, your noticing is still followed by eating. The pattern of following your thoughts into the kitchen may be deeply entrenched. Fortunately, if you're patient and vigilant, noticing these food thoughts will eventually lead to being able to ignore them.

Frozen Fruit

Frozen Grapes

Nutritional Info:
Servings Per Recipe: 1
Amount Per Serving
Calories: 95.7
Total Fat: 0.2 g
Cholesterol: 0.0 mg
Sodium: 2.8 mg
Total Carbs: 24.8 g
Dietary Fiber: 0.9 g
Protein: 0.9 g

Ingredients:
grapes

Directions:
Remove grapes from stems and freeze for 24 hours
.

Frozen Banana

Nutritional Info:
Servings Per Recipe: 1
Amount Per Serving
Calories: 108.5
Total Fat: 0.6 g
Cholesterol: 0.0 mg
Sodium: 1.2 mg
Total Carbs: 27.7 g
Dietary Fiber: 2.8 g
Protein: 1.2 g

Ingredients:
One medium banana

Directions: Freeze. Eat frozen.

Orange Slices

Nutritional Info:
Servings Per Recipe: 1
Amount Per Serving
Calories: 61.6
Total Fat: 0.1 g
Cholesterol: 0.0 mg
Sodium: 0.0 mg
Total Carbs: 15.4 g
Dietary Fiber: 3.1 g
Protein: 1.2 g

Ingredients:
One medium orange

Directions: Freeze. Eat frozen.

Frozen Cherries

Nutritional Info:
Servings Per Recipe: 1
Amount Per Serving
Calories: 73.7
Total Fat: 0.2 g
Cholesterol: 0.0 mg
Sodium: 0.0 mg
Total Carbs: 18.7 g
Dietary Fiber: 2.5 g
Protein: 1.2 g

Ingredients:
Frozen Cherries

Directions: Freeze. Eat frozen.

Kung Fu for Cravings and Emotional Eating

Have you ever had a feeling of gnawing, insatiable emptiness that just won't let go of you? That is what I felt when I was on the verge of an emotional-eating attack. Something or someone was bugging me, and all I wanted to do was stuff myself with the best-tasting food I could find. I wasn't picky at this point. I just *needed* to eat something, pronto! This feeling of urgency was so strong because I'd followed it and reinforced it over and over for years.

Eating was how I coped with life. If life didn't feel good, I indulged in negative thoughts that made me feel even worse. To feel better, I ate too much. If stress or an uncomfortable emotion came on the scene, my hand automatically reached for food, and I turned into an eating machine. Happiness was the issue and eating a mere symptom.

Emotional eating is eating without being completely aware that you're eating. Instead, you're thinking and feeling—and feeding your feelings with—stressful thoughts while semi-consciously shoveling down copious quantities of food, perhaps without even tasting it.

If this has been your habit, the compulsion to eat feels so strong that it seems physical. The strength of the compulsion is actually due to the countless times you've reinforced it by reaching for food to soothe uncomfortable emotions. But fear not! It's possible to interrupt this pattern, and the list of powerful kung fu exercises below can help.

Banana Yogurt Sauce

Nutritional Info
Servings Per Recipe: 2
Amount Per Serving
Calories: 150.3
Total Fat: 0.3 g
Cholesterol: 0.0 mg
Sodium: 65.8 mg
Total Carbs: 21.1 g
Dietary Fiber: 1.4 g
Protein: 15.6 g

Ingredients:
Fage Greek Yogurt 0% fat, 12 oz
Banana, fresh, 1 medium (7" to 7-7/8" long)
Vanilla Extract, 1 tsp

Directions:
Place all ingredients in a blender. Blend on a medium speed and
serve.

Powerful Kung Fu #1: Dis-identify with the Feeling

1. Notice that a craving is on the scene and get yourself the heck out of the kitchen!
2. Ask yourself, "What am I feeling right now?" Wait for the answer.
3. When the answer comes, ask yourself, "**What is noticing [the particular feeling you are feeling]?**" Fill in the blank with whatever feeling is present. Let's say agitation is present. Ask yourself, "What is noticing agitation?" This question helps you dis-identify with the feeling.

Or

Say to yourself, "**It's just [the particular feeling]. What a relief. It's not me. It couldn't be me because I'm over here, noticing it.**" It's such a huge relief to realize that the feeling is not you! Normally we merge with negative feelings and assume they're *our* feelings, but they belong to the ego, not to us—not to who we really are. When we identify with the feeling, we have little power or objectivity. But when we notice a feeling, we're outside of it, aligned with the Wise Witness. In my experience, this kung fu cuts the power of the feeling in half immediately.

Apple Pecan Bread

Nutritional Info:
Servings Per Recipe: 16
Amount Per Serving
Calories: 183.9
Total Fat: 8.8 g
Cholesterol: 115.0 mg
Sodium: 284.8 mg
Total Carbs: 23.8 g
Dietary Fiber: 3.7 g
Protein: 5.1 g

Ingredients:
oat flour, 2 2/3 cups
Cinnamon, ground, 2 tsp
Salt, 1 tsp
Baking Soda, 1.5 tsp
Nutmeg, ground, 1.5 tsp
Egg, fresh, 4 large
Vanilla Extract, 2 tsp
Walnuts, 1 cup, chopped
Apples, fresh, 4 cup, quartered or chopped
Banana, fresh, 4 medium (7" to 7-7/8" long)
Butter, salted, melted, 1 tbsp

Directions:
Combine all ingredients and place in a greased non-stick pan (you may also use parchment paper to prevent sticking). Bake at 325 degrees for 20 minutes. Keep testing with a toothpick every five minutes and remove from the oven when the toothpick comes out clean.

Powerful Kung Fu #2: Allow the Feeling to Be There

1. Notice that a craving is on the scene and get yourself the heck out of the kitchen!
2. Drop your story about the feeling and simply allow it to be there. Notice the sensation. What does it feel like in your body? Allow the feeling to be there without any agenda for it to dissipate. Accepting it and allowing it to be present will enable it to eventually dissolve. Emotions don't come to stay; they come to leave. If you can learn to stop feeding them with more negative thoughts, they dissolve more quickly. The best internal posture is simply to be present and allow whatever is happening in the moment, without adding more negative thoughts to it. Ask yourself, **"Can I just allow [the particular feeling] to be here?"**

Vanilla Pudding

Preparation Time:
10 minutes (excluding the cooking time for the rice and sweet potatoes)

Nutritional Info:
Servings Per Recipe: 6
Amount Per Serving
Calories: 153.8
Total Fat: 1.0 g
Cholesterol: 0.0 mg
Sodium: 235.1 mg
Total Carbs: 31.2 g
Dietary Fiber: 3.3 g
Protein: 3.5 g

Ingredients:
Salt, 1 t
Pure Vanilla Extract 1 T
Sweet Potato Cooked 1 ½ cups
Cooked Brown Rice, medium grain, 2 cups (can use Trader Joe's frozen organic brown rice thawed)
Low Fat Vanilla Soy Milk, 1 cup

Directions:
Blend in a food processor or blender and serve.

Powerful Kung Fu #3: Identify the Need

1. Notice that a craving is on the scene and get yourself the heck out of the kitchen!
2. Ask yourself, **"What am I needing right now that is causing me to want some pleasure?"**
3. If the answer is appreciation, comfort, or understanding, in your imagination, give yourself what you need—a hug or words of consolation or praise.
4. Alternatively, ask yourself, **"Is there something else here that's whole and complete and doesn't need anything?"** This will help you see the real you, the you that doesn't actually need what you may think you need.

Chocolate (or Carob) Pudding

Preparation Time:
10 minutes (excluding the cooking time for the rice and sweet potatoes)

Nutritional Info:
Servings Per Recipe: 6
Amount Per Serving
Calories: 186.6
Total Fat: 3.0 g
Cholesterol: 0.0 mg
Sodium: 238.1 mg
Total Carbs: 38.9 g
Dietary Fiber: 8.1 g
Protein: 6.3 g

Nutritional Info: (with walnuts)
Servings Per Recipe: 6
Amount Per Serving
Calories: 210.6
Total Fat: 7.5 g
Cholesterol: 0.0 mg
Sodium: 227.9 mg
Total Carbs: 30.8 g
Dietary Fiber: 3.8 g
Protein: 4.7 g

Ingredients:
Salt, 1 t
Pure Vanilla Extract 1 T
Sweet Potato Cooked 1½ cups
Cooked Brown Rice, medium grain, 2 cups (can use Trader Joe's frozen organic brown rice thawed)
Low Fat Vanilla Soy Milk, 1 cup
Cocoa or Carob, dry powder, unsweetened, 1 cup or 4 squares of unsweetened baking chocolate
Walnuts, 1/2 cup, chopped (optional)

Directions:
Blend in a food processor or blender and serve.

Powerful Kung Fu #4: Is There Something I Need to Address?

1. Notice that a craving is on the scene and get yourself the heck out of the kitchen!
2. Ask yourself, **"Is there something I need to address inside myself, with another person, or in my life?"** Get curious about what that could be and be prepared for insights to arise. Then, take action to address any disharmonies or imbalances.

Lemon Pudding

Preparation Time:
10 minutes (excluding the cooking time for the rice and sweet potatoes)

Nutritional Info:
Servings Per Recipe: 6
Amount Per Serving
Calories: 146.4
Total Fat: 0.9 g
Cholesterol: 0.0 mg
Sodium: 227.8 mg
Total Carbs: 30.3 g
Dietary Fiber: 3.2 g
Protein: 3.2 g

Ingredients:
Salt, 1 t
Pure Vanilla Extract 1 T
Sweet Potato Cooked 1 ½ cups
Cooked Brown Rice, medium grain, 2 cups (can use Trader Joe's frozen organic brown rice thawed)
Low Fat Vanilla Soy Milk, 1 cup
Lemon Juice ¼ cup

Directions:
Blend in a food processor or blender and serve.

Powerful Kung Fu #5: Dis-identify with the Troublesome Food Thought

1. Notice that a craving is on the scene and get yourself the heck out of the kitchen!
2. Ask yourself, "What is it that is aware of the thought 'I want food right now'?
3. Next, ask, "Is that thought or impulse to eat really me? If I am aware of it, how can it be me?" Once you realize that this thought is not you, you automatically dis-identify with it, and it loses its power.

Powerful Kung Fu #6: The Mosquito Flick

1. Notice that a craving is on the scene and get yourself the heck out of the kitchen!
2. Notice that an impractical food thought is on the scene and imagine flicking it away, the same way you would flick away an annoying mosquito.

Apple Cinnamon Walnut Pudding

Preparation Time:
15 minutes (excluding the cooking time for the rice and sweet potatoes)

Nutritional Info:
Servings Per Recipe: 6
Amount Per Serving
Calories: 305.1
Total Fat: 14.4 g
Cholesterol: 0.0 mg
Sodium: 229.2 mg
Total Carbs: 39.3 g
Dietary Fiber: 6.1 g
Protein: 6.4 g

Ingredients:
Salt, 1 t
Pure Vanilla Extract 1 T
Sweet Potato Cooked 1½ cups
Cooked Brown Rice, medium grain, 2 cups (can use Trader Joe's frozen organic brown rice thawed)
Low Fat Vanilla Soy Milk, 1 cup
Apples, fresh, 2 cup, peeled, quartered or chopped
Walnuts, 1 cup, chopped
Cinnamon, ground, 2 tsp

Directions:
Blend in a food processor or blender and serve.

Powerful Kung Fu #7: Notice that the Child Is on the Scene

1. Notice that a craving is on the scene and get yourself the heck out of the kitchen!
2. Tell yourself, "Oh, that's just the Child. No big deal. For a minute there, I thought I wanted to eat something, but it was just what the Child wanted. She wanted to distract me. Thank goodness it's just the Child and not me."

Apple Cinnamon Raisin Pudding

Preparation Time:
15 minutes (excluding the cooking time for the rice and sweet potatoes)

Nutritional Info:
Servings Per Recipe: 6
Amount Per Serving
Calories: 243.0
Total Fat: 1.2 g
Cholesterol: 0.0 mg
Sodium: 230.8 mg
Total Carbs: 55.5 g
Dietary Fiber: 5.6 g
Protein: 4.1 g

Ingredients:
Salt, 1 t
Pure Vanilla Extract 1 T
Sweet Potato Cooked 1½ cups
Cooked Brown Rice, medium grain, 2 cups (can use Trader Joe's frozen organic brown rice thawed)
Low Fat Vanilla Soy Milk, 1 cup
Raisins, fresh, 1 cup
Walnuts, 1 cup, chopped
Cinnamon, ground, 2 t

Directions:
Blend in a food processor or blender and serve.

Powerful Kung Fu #8: See the Whole Picture of Food

1. Notice that a craving is on the scene and get yourself the heck out of the kitchen!
2. Remember the whole picture of food. The pleasure of eating a particular food is so short-lived! Imagine how bad you will feel if you overeat—the shame, blame, self-castigation, bloating, long term health impact, possible weight gain, irritability, etc.

Peanut Butter Banana Pudding

Preparation Time:
15 minutes (excluding the cooking time for the rice and sweet potatoes)

Nutritional Info:
Servings Per Recipe: 6
Amount Per Serving
Calories: 274.2
Total Fat: 9.1 g
Cholesterol: 0.0 mg
Sodium: 305.8 mg
Total Carbs: 42.1 g
Dietary Fiber: 5.4 g
Protein: 7.4 g

Ingredients:
Salt, 1 t
Pure Vanilla Extract 1 T
Sweet Potato Cooked 1½ cups
Cooked Brown Rice, medium grain, 2 cups (can use Trader Joe's frozen organic brown rice thawed)
Low Fat Vanilla Soy Milk, 1 cup
Banana, fresh, 2 medium (7" to 7-7/8" long)
Peanut Butter, chunk style, 6 tbsp

Directions:
Blend in a food processor or blender and serve.

Powerful Kung Fu #9: Put Your Attention on Something Else

1. Notice that a craving is on the scene and get yourself the heck out of the kitchen!
2. Do or think about something else. Read a book. Talk to someone. Take a walk. Do a crossword puzzle. Finish the laundry. Drive somewhere. Turn on the television. Listen to music. Meditate. Focus on your senses. What are you feeling, seeing, smelling, or hearing? Almost any distraction will do. Make a list of noneating activities you find engaging and nurturing so that when a craving strikes, you're ready for it.
3. Don't give your attention to ego-based thoughts (especially negative ones), thoughts that are about "me" or "my story" or that start with "I," such as "I like, I want, I don't want, I hope, I don't like, I feel, I think, I believe, I can't, I won't, I'm not, I did..." This involvement with the "me" is what gave you the craving crazies in the first place.

Oatmeal Raisin Cookies

Nutritional Info:
Servings Per Recipe: 8
Amount Per Serving
Calories: 137.0
Total Fat: 3.0 g
Cholesterol: 30.4 mg
Sodium: 207.9 mg
Total Carbs: 30.4 g
Dietary Fiber: 3.1 g
Protein: 3.0 g

Ingredients:
Oats, .75 cup)
Baking Soda, .25 tsp
Cinnamon, ground, .5 tsp
Salt, .5 tsp
Egg, fresh, 1 large
Raisins, 1 cup (not packed)
Sweet potato, 1 cup, cubes
Butter, salted, 1 tbsp
Vanilla Extract, 2 tsp
oat flour, 0.25 cup

Directions: Blend by hand. Preheat oven to 325 degrees. For cookies scoop out in using teaspoons and place on a cookie sheet coated with baking spray. Bake for 15 minutes, longer if you like them crisper. For bars spread in a Pyrex pan coated with cooking spray. Bake for 20-30 minutes depending on how firm you like them.

Powerful Kung Fu #10: Get Engaged in What You're Doing

1. Notice that a craving is on the scene and get yourself the heck out of the kitchen!
2. Become engaged and focus completely on whatever you're doing now, whether it's work, running an errand, vacuuming, finishing a good book, or making a call. When you're really absorbed in something, you can go for hours without a single thought about food.